Keto Diet for Beginners 2018:

Start Your Fat Burning Weight Loss Journey!

Randall Colbert

ISBN: 9781726860666

CONTENTS

INTRODUCTION

If you haven't been living under a rock for the past year, you may have heard of the keto diet. You're probably asking the question "what can a keto diet for me?". This book is designed to answer just that. But before answering that question, let's take a little tour of what this book covers and dive into the history of the keto diet.

This book is not a cookbook, it is a book about the keto diet and how it can benefit your body and metal wellbeing. That's not to say it will not have any dietary advice, rest assured, it will. This book will cover the following:

- What is the Keto Diet

- What kind of foods to eat

- Why you should eat keto

- How to get into ketosis

- How you know you're in ketosis

- Tips about staying in ketosis

- Side effects of the keto diet

- Foods to avoid on a keto diet

- Foods to eat on a keto diet

The keto diet is not a recent phenomenon, it was popularized in the 1920s and 30s as a way to treat epilepsy. However, the diet was later abandoned thanks to new antiepileptic drugs emerging.

The idea of fasting to treat diseases has been know for thousands of years and was studied in great detail by ancient Greek and Indian physicians. But the first modern study for using fasting as a cure for epilepsy was carried out in 1911, in France. During these times epileptics were treated using potassium bromide. During the study, it was discovered that fasting showed much greater results in the patients cognitive function, when compared to taking potassium bromide.

THE KETO DIET

What exactly is the keto diet? The keto in ketogenic diet comes from the fact that the body produces molecules called ketones which can be used to fuel the body. Ketones are used as an alternative fuel source when you body runs short on blood sugar, also known as glucose.

So when you deprive your body from carbohydrates, your body resorts to using ketones as its primary source of fuel. Ketones are produced in the liver from fats. They are then sent to all your body organs, including the brain to be used for energy. The most hungry organ in your body is the brain, which means it's unable be getting its energy from only fats. It needs to get the energy from either glucose or ketones.

When you're on a ketogenic diet, your entire body runs almost entirely on fat. This means a lot of fat is burned as it get used up for energy and insulin levels run very low. This is why a ketogenic diet is so great if you're trying to lose fat. You burn fat by just doing day to day activities. Your body burns fat without you even doing anything. There's also the added benefit of being less hungry thanks to having access to a steady supply of energy. You'll also find that when you're on a ketogenic diet you become much more focused and alert.

When you're on a keto diet, your goal is to keep you body in a state known as ketosis. When your body is in ketosis, it's producing ketones as it's primary source of energy. The fastest way to get into a state of ketosis is by fasting, but nobody can fast forever. This is where the keto diet comes to the rescue.

A keto diet allows you to stay in a constant state of ketosis without dieting. It has many of the same benefits that fasting does, without the downside of not eating anything.

A keto diet is safe, but you should consult a doctor if you fall under any of the following conditions.

- Do you take medication for diabetes, such as insulin?

- Do you take medication for high blood pressure?

- Do you breastfeed?

If any of the these conditions apply to you
then take special consideration when going on
a keto diet.

WHAT IS KETOSIS

So what exactly is ketosis? To put it simply, ketosis is when your body is fueled by fat and ketones instead of just glucose. This has the benefit of burning fat and increasing cognitive function.

Ok so we know what ketosis is, but what are ketones? It's a common misconception that the brain needs carbohydrates to fuel itself. But carbs are not the only fuel your brain is able to run off of. If you consume a lot of carbs then yes, your brain will use that as its fuel source, but when you avoid carbs your brain is just as happy to use ketones as its fuel source.

Using ketones as a fuel source for your brain is absolutely necessary for survival. Your body can only store enough carbohydrates to last for one or two days. If it wasn't for ketones, your brain will quickly shut down as soon as those carbohydrates stores run out. Back when food wasn't available all day every day, humans entered a state of ketosis regularly. But in the modern age there's always food available, so ketosis has now become extremely rare.

Our bodies have evolved a way to use fats stores as energy. This means we can go days, if not weeks without eating anything. Ketones is what allows our brain to run on those fat stores too.

So the bottom line is that we don't need carbohydrates at all. The brain can happily run on fat thanks to ketones.

Many people have experienced that their brain runs much better on ketones than it does glucose. People feel energized, happier and more focused when on a keto diet. Fat loss is the cherry on top.

BENEFITS OF KETOSIS

There are many benefits when entering a state of ketosis. When you enter ketosis, your body is given an almost unlimited supply of energy that can help increase your cognitive and physical abilities. Weight loss will also become effortless and you'll find yourself losing weight without even doing much exercise.

Ketosis has a long history of being used to treat illnesses such as epilepsy. By entering ketosis, you're effectively doing the opposite of type 2 diabetes.

Let's list a few of the benefits that a keto diet has to offer.

<u>Appetite Control</u>

When you're in ketosis, you'll find that you have the new found power to control your appetite. This is thanks to the fact that your body is constantly burning fat for energy, giving you a constant supply of energy which means reduced feelings of hunger.

Being able to control your appetite means you'll find it much easier to eat less, thus making losing weight effortless. You simply won't feel like eating unless you're truly hungry. This has the added benefit of saving money as you won't feel the need to buy any snacks. People have often experienced the need to only eat twice a day, sometimes even once a day.

Having control of your appetite also helps with addiction to junk foods and eating disorders such as bulimia. You can still enjoy food, but you'll start seeing it as more of a friend and not an enemy.

Weight Loss

Your body will transform into a lean, mean, fat burning machine. When you're in a state of ketosis your body will constantly be burning fat to supply energy to every muscle and organ in your body. Your insulin hormone levels will drop dramatically, creating the ideal fat losing environment for your body. There are many scientific studies that show that a low carb keto diet will result in extremely effective weight loss.

Increased Cognitive Function

When your body is in ketosis, you gain access to a steady stream of energy to your body and brain. This means you will avoid big swings in blood sugar levels. Which in turn leads to a heightened sense of focus and concentration. No longer will you experience foggy memory. Many people go on the keto diet specifically for the benefit of increased cognitive function. In fact, the keto diet is popular among elite chess players.

When you're on the keto diet, your brain stops relying on carbs for energy. It instead runs on ketones, the ultimate fuel source for your brain.

Quite Stomach

The keto diet has been documented to result in less gas, cramps and stomach pains. This can be a very important reason to switch to a keto diet if you experience chronic stomach upsets. People have noticed a difference in less than two days!

If you sufferer from irritable bowel syndrome (IBS) you might want to consider going on a keto diet. It's very common for a keto diet to dramatically improve IBS symptoms.

Improved Overall Health

Many studies have shown that a keto diet improves important health markers such as blood sugar levels, insulin levels, blood pressure and cholesterol.

Increased Endurance

Your endurance will skyrocket thanks to the constant supply of energy your body gets by burning fat. Your bodies supply of stored carbohydrates, known as glycogen only lasts for a couple of hours during intense exercise. But your fat reserves will last much, much longer.

When your body is used to using carbohydrates as a fuel source, your fat reserves will rarely be used so it can't fuel the brain. This means you always have to eat your fill to replenish your bodies supply of carbohydrates during or after an intense exercise. But when you're on a ketogenic diet your brain and body are constantly fueled by fat and ketones. You will feel like you're able to go on forever.

It's a common misconception that carbohydrates are needed to perform exercise. Your body can perform physical exercise perfectly fine when burning fat for energy. But you need to remember the following two points in order to not suffer from reduced performance.

- Take enough fluids and salts. When you're taking a low carb diet, it's extremely important to take enough fluids and salt. Drink a glass of water with half a tea spoon of salt an hour before exercise. This will dramatically increase your performance.

- It takes some time for your body to get used to ketosis. Your body will need at least two week to get used to the transition of using glucose as its primary source of energy to using fat and ketones as it's primary source of energy. The more you exercise on a low carb diet, the quicker your body will get used to using fat and ketones to fuel the body.

When you first start exercising on a keto diet you may notice reduced performance. But fear not, as this will only be temporary and you will see many benefits in the long term. The idea of using a low carb diet for increased physical performance is quite a recent phenomenon and many athletes are just now starting to experiment with it. The benefits of a low carb diet are mainly seen in sports of endurance, such as long running. Your bodies far reserves hold much greater energy potential than your bodies glycogen stores. This means once you've transitioned to using fat for energy instead of glycogen, you will experience less fatigue and find yourself being able to perform much longer without the need for any additional food for fuel.

Your body won't have to fuel any gastrointestinal organ activity during physical activity. This means more blood will flow to your working muscles resulting in greater physical performance.

One of the side effects of a keto diet is that your body will have a very low fat percentage which can be a huge benefit for many sports.

<u>Help with Epilepsy</u>
The keto diet is a tried and tested method to treat epilepsy. It has been used since the 1920s to treat children, but has recently seen benefits to treating adults too. There are a multitude of studies done that show that a keto diet is one of the most effective ways to treat epilepsy. When you're on a keto diet

while suffering from epilepsy you'll be able to reduce the amount of anti-epileptic drugs you take and still remain seizure free. This means all the side effects from taking anti-epileptic drugs such as drowsiness, reduced concentration and IQ are gone. It's still important to consult your doctor before going off of medication.

Controlled Blood Sugar

The keto diet has been shown to control blood sugar levels and even reverse type 2 diabetes. This is because its been shown to reduce blood sugar levels as well as soften the negative impact of high insulin levels.

Because the keto diet restricts carbohydrates, your body will use fats for fuel instead of sugar, so naturally your blood sugar level will fall dramatically.

Acne

Acne is extremely common in adolescents and teens but it's also fairly common in adults as well. It's estimated that roughly 50% of adults aged between 20 and 30 struggle from acne.

Acne develops when the gland on your skin that produces oil to lubricate your skin and hair becomes impaired. Increased levels of hormones known as androgens causes increased oil production which leads to oily skin, resulting in dead skin cells not shedding effectively. This causes blocks in the pores of the skin.

Like your gut, your skin also has its own microbiome with an ecosystem of bacteria. One kind of bacteria, P. Acnes resides within hair follicles, but during acne the level of P. Acnes increases dramatically which causes inflammation and white heads.

It was thought that diets high in sugar and refined carbs caused acne. However, in the 1960s experiments showed that diet didn't actually contribute much to causing acne. But now the tides have turned and recent research within the past decade has shown that diets high in carbohydrates do in fact have an effect on acne. This is because high carb diets have a negative effect on your bodies ability to regulate hormones. In 2007 a study was carried out by Robyn N Smith on acne prone men. In this study, it was found that a low glycemic diet led to a greater reduction in acne lesions than a high glycemic diet. In addition, it was found that the group that took the low glycemic diet experienced lower insulin and androgen levels while also losing weight. In contrast, the group that took the high glycemic diet experienced weight gain and increased insulin and androgen levels.

In 2012 Italian researchers discussed potential benefits that a keto diet can have in regards to acne. The following benefits could help in reducing acne:

- Reduced Insulin Levels: High Insulin levels causes an increased production of skin cells, sebum and androgen, all of which increases the likelihood of an acne breakout. A keto diet will dramatically decrease insulin levels.

- Anti-Inflammatory: Inflammation only makes acne worse. Keto diets have been shown to greatly reduce the effects of inflammation

- Decreased levels of IGF-1, an insulin growth factor. Like insulin, IGF-1 increases sebum production and has been found to play a large role in the development of acne.

Less Migraine

While migraines and epilepsy are separate medical issues, they are both neurological brain disorders and often require similar medication. People with migraine may experience less attacks. The reason for this is somewhat of a mystery, but many people have claimed it has helped with migraine. Researchers speculate that it might be something to do with the reduced blood sugar and insulin that comes with a keto diet, but this is still being researched.

Less Heartburn

Heartburn is very common, millions of people suffer from it around the world. Many people resort to medication to reduce the everyday symptoms of it. But what if these people could cure this disease with a dietary change?

Early, small tests were done that put sufferers of heart disease on a low carb, high fat diet. The patients got significantly better and even saw improved pH levels in the esophagus. A recent larger study was done and tested this idea once again. They found a link between carbohydrates, sugar and glycogen. They all contributed to reflux disease. They also found that participates that were on a low carb, high fat diet were able to go off their reflux medication without any negative side effects.

Reduced Sugar Cravings

Because a keto diet has little to no sweeteners, you will see a significantly reduced craving for sugar while also staying satisfied. In addition you'll also get all the other benefits a keto diet comes with, which includes weight loss and enhanced physical and metal performance.

Alzheimer's Preventions

The brain loves ketones. As previously discussed, your brain gets its fuel from two sources, which are ketones and glucose. But ketones are a much better fuel source than glucose. Ketones are produced when fat is broken down into fatty acids. There is evidence that suggests that certain brain functions can improve by using ketones for brain fuels instead of glucose. Ever since it was discovered that a keto diet can help cure epilepsy, there have been a number of researchers finding ways a keto diet can help other brain disorders. While the exact mechanisms behind ketones and brain health are unclear, ketones have been shown to increase mitochondrial respiration, which results in more energy production, increased neurological growth, reduced brain inflammation and reduced oxidative stress.

When somebody suffers from Alzheimer's, the brain becomes resistant to insulin, which results in less efficiency when using glucose as a fuel source. This has been very well documented, in fact some researchers have come to call Alzheimer's type 3 diabetes. The fact that this insulin resistance reduces the ability for the brain to use glucose helps explain the higher rates of Alzheimer's in people that are diabetic.

Insulin resistance can even effect people who aren't diabetic and people who are years away from any mental symptoms. People who are prediabetic and young women with polycystic ovarian syndrome can also suffer from insulin resistance of the brain. A low carb diet such as the keto diet can help with this problem. This is because with a keto diet, the brain won't be receiving it's fuel from glucose anyway, and instead receive it's fuel from ketones. When somebody suffers form Alzheimer's disease, the brain ability to metabolize glucose can fall as much as 40%, this gap in energy increases the risk of neurological dysfunction and neurological decline.

The scientific rationale for using ketones for Alzheimer's is solid, but it's still seen as an unorthodox approach by many Alzheimer's researchers. There have only been a small number of Human clinical trial, but here is a summary of those trials.

- The first trial was done in 2004 by a group of Japanese researchers. They took 19 healthy adults with no mental disorders and were over the age 60. These participants were fed on a keto diet. It was found that those that scored the lowest in a cognitive test prior to going on a keto diet showed the most improvement in terms of visual attention, memory and task switching.

- A study led by US researcher Dr. Robert Krikorian assigned 23 adults with mild cognitive impairment to either six weeks on a low carb keto diet or a high carb, low fat diet. The participants that were on a keto diet lost weight and saw improvements in their blood sugar and insulin levels. Memory performance was also tested and it was found that those on a keto diet showed improvements. The participants with the greatest improvement were those that had the highest levels of ketones in the blood.

- In 2017, a team of researchers from Kansas published the results of their studies on the feasibility of the keto diet to treat Alzheimer's. In this study, 15 participants with Alzheimer's were put on a ketogenic diet for three months. A family member was required to cook for them for those months, but four participants dropped out because the task was to burdensome for the care givers. 10 out of 11 of the remaining participants saw an average of a 4.1 point improvement in cognitive tests. A month after going off the diet, these cognitive improvements were lost.

Treatment For Brain Cancer

The premise of using a keto diet to treat cancer falls on the fact that cancer needs glucose to fuel their rapid growth. In fact, this is precisely how PET scans diagnose cancer. An injection of radioactive sugar illuminates the cancer cells because they require much more glucose than your typical non-cancerous cell to fuel their rapid growth. Cancer cell growth can also be fueled by glutamine, which is an amino acid created from the breakdown of proteins.

By starving cancer from their fuel source and using ketones instead to fuel the cells is the conceptual theory behind using a ketogenic diet as a way to treat cancer. Ordinary cells have the ability to switch between using ketones and glucose for energy, cancer cells do not. The chronic starvation of the fuel they need to grow stresses and weakens the cancer cells. Which makes them much more vulnerable to treatments such as chemotherapy, radiation or hyperbaric oxygen.

The keto diet is particularly effective against cancer cells when combined with periods of intermittent fasting. When fasting, ketone production is increased which makes it easier to starve cancer cells. Today's modern diet promotes snacking and has us eating up to five meals a day, preventing any sort of intermittent fasting. When nutrition is being constantly supplied , blood sugar and insulin levels remain high. The fuel source to allow cancer to grow and develop is constantly available.

A fasting lifestyle involves eating for a period of only 4-8 hours in one day. A 20 hour fast might involve eating between 3pm and 7pm each day. This intermittent fasting lifestyle increase the production of ketones by your body.

HOW TO GET INTO KETOSIS

There are many things you can do to get your body to enter ketosis. The following is a list of ways for you to get into ketosis, listed from most important to least.

Restrict Carbohydrates

The main thing you need to focus on is to restrict the amount of carbohydrates entering your body. Ideally, you'll limit yourself to 20 grams of carbs or less a day. Even though fiber is a carbohydrate it does not need to be restricted as it's undigestible, in fact keeping fiber in your diet can be beneficial. Here is a list of foods that are very low in carbs.

Meat – No amount of carbs
Fish – No amount of carbs
Olive Oil – No amount of carbs
Coconut Fat – No amount of carbs
Butter – Very low in carbs
Eggs – 1 Egg contains less than 1 gram of carbs
Avocado – Very low in carbs
Cheese – Low in carbs

Consume Proteins at a Moderate Level

When you're on a keto diet, you should only eat the proteins you need and not much more. This is because any excess protein gets converted into glucose, which you don't want in your system because it will cause your body do use less ketones for fuel. You should aim to stay at or below 1 gram of protein a day per body weight. So if your weigh 80kg, you should aim to consume 80 grams of protein a day or less. Too much protein consumption is one of the most common reasons that stop people from entering ketosis.

Eat Enough Fat

You'll want to eat enough fat until you're satisfied. You must remember there's a huge difference between a keto diet and starvation. A keto diet is sustainable, whereas starvation is not. When you're starving you feel tired and low energy, but a keto diet will make you feel great and give you plenty of energy. So you should eat until you're full. If you still feel hungry while on a keto diet, it could be a sign that you're not getting enough fat. Some good sources of fat that include little to no carbs are:

- Butter
- Olive Oil
- Coconut Oil
- Mayonnaise
- Heavy Cream
- Guacamole

Avoid Snacking

Eating just for the sake of eating when you're not hungry reduces the effects of ketosis and also leads to weight gain. But if you really can't give up snacking, then keto friendly snacks will be the best option for you. Some quick keto friendly snacks that take little to no time to prepare are:

- Eggs
- Cheese
- Avocado
- Cold cut meat
- Olives
- Macadamia, Pecan and Brazil nuts

These snacks have minimal carbohydrates and are packed with plenty of healthy fats.

Prefer more vegetarian oriented snacks? These snacks also have low amounts of carbohydrates and are suitable for vegetarians

- Celery
- Cucumber
- Red, green and yellow peppers
- Carrot
- Cream cheese, sour cream or any high fat dipping sauce.

Craving for something more juicy? These berries go great with a topping of heavy whipped cream:

- Raspberry
- Blackberry
- Strawberry

Berries can be a great snack to have from time to time. But be careful not to have too many as that can take you out of ketosis. The best berries to have are Raspberry, followed by blackberries and strawberries as these have the lowest amount of carbs. Blueberries should be avoided as they have a high number of carbs compared to the previously mentioned berries.

You may be surprised, but chocolate can be

eaten occasionally on a keto diet. But keep your consumption to a minimum, one or two squares at most. Avoid dark or milk chocolate as these are too high in carbs. High cocoa chocolates between 70 and 90 percent are the best options.

Some other keto friendly snacks include:

Pork Rinds – Also known as pork crisps or cracklings, pork rinds are a tasty snacks with no carbs.

Beef Jerky – Some commercially sold beef jerky may contain high amounts of sugar, so be sure to check the packaging before purchasing.

Biltong - A dried spiced meat that originates from South Africa. Usually made of beef, ostrich or venison. This is meat that's marinated in salt, vinegar and spices for a few days and then dried. Typically low in sugar.

People make a lot of mistakes when it comes to snacking on a keto diet. Some foods have surprisingly high amounts of carbohydrates, here is a list of some seemingly ordinary foods that are packed with carbohydrates. Some of these foods may come at a surprise.

- **Grapes** – 1 bunch of grapes equates to 16 grams of carbs
- **Bananas** – 20 grams of carbs
- **Caffe Latte** – 18 grams of carbs
- **Cashew nuts** – 27 grams of carbs per serving
- **Vitamin Water** – 32 grams of carbs per 20 oz bottle
- **Fruit Juice** – 32 grams of carbs per 20 oz glass

When you're on a keto diet, there are snacks that you must avoid at all costs. These snacks hold little to no nutritional value, are packed with carbohydrates and are just plain unhealthy. Common snacking foods like donuts, chips, candy and most chocolate bars are a no go. Do not eat them if you're on a keto diet and you want to go into ketosis. The good news is that once you're on a keto diet, your cravings for junk food will quickly go away. Be very wary of sweet foods that are marketed as being keto friendly, if you eat these foods you run the risk of developing a craving for sugary foods which can lead you to eat more than you need.

Sometimes you just want a quick bite to eat before dinner, here are some quick and easy to make snacks that are tasty and keto friendly.

- Slice of cheese with celery, cucumber, radish or wrapped in lettuce

- Celery filled with cream cheese, natural peanut butter, brie or other soft cheese

- Slice of cheese smeared with butter

- Cucumber or lettuce spread with mayo

- Parmesan crisps smeared with butter

- Slice of salami and cheese, rolled together

- Slice of bacon smeared with peanut butter

- Piece of dark chocolate smeared with butter

- Shot glass of heavy cream

- Spoonful of crème fraiche

- Spoonful of butter, ghee or coconut oil melted into coffee or tea

Intermitted Fasting

If you're finding it difficult to go into ketosis, try doing some intermitted fasting. For example, you could skip breakfast and only eat in 8 hour periods, fasting for 16 hours. This is popular way to fast and is known as 8:16 fasting. It can lead to weight loss and even the reversal of type 2 to diabetes. Intermitted fasting is also a lot easier to do when you're on a keto diet as your body will be accustomed to burning fat for energy.

Exercise

Performing any physical activity while on a keto diet will enhance ketone production moderately. While exercise is not necessary to enter ketosis, it can prove to be helpful in increasing ketone levels and has the added benefit of helping you to lose weight.

Get Enough Sleep

Most people need at least seven hours of sleep

every night. When you become sleep deprived, your stress hormone levels and blood sugar levels rise considerably. This slows down ketosis and makes it much harder to stick to a keto diet. While getting enough sleep alone is not enough to get you into ketosis, it can prove to be very beneficial in keeping you onto a keto diet and helping you resist temptations.

In summary, to get into a keto diet, the number one most important thing to do is to restrict carbohydrates. You want to be taking a maximum of 20 grams of carbs a day. This is extremely important to enter and maintain ketosis. If you still need help entering ketosis, you can take additional measures by looking into the previously listed steps.

The great thing about ketosis is that it's completely natural, there's no need for expensive supplements, such as MTC oil and ketone supplements. There's no evidence that any of these supplements even work, so there's no need for them. Ketone supplements do not lower insulin or blood sugar levels, neither do they enhance fat burning. Your body can produce its own ketones naturally and it's very good at doing so.

People that claim supplements do help them, most likely do so for financial reasons. They might tell you that there product is fantastic and that it'll change your life, but like all other miracle supplements, this is hardly the case. So take those stories with a grain of salt.
That's not to say these supplements do nothing at all. Taking ketone supplements will raise your ketone levels, but these effects are temporary and will only last for a few hours.

HOW TO KNOW WHEN YOU'RE IN KETOSIS

So you're on a keto diet, but how do you know when you're actually in ketosis? Well there are actually a few ways to know. It's possible to find out by testing urine, blood or breath samples but there are also symptoms you experience that help let you know when you're in a state of ketosis.

One of the symptoms you might get is a dry mouth and feelings of thirst. Unless you drink a lot of water and get enough electrolytes, such as salt, your mouth may feel dry. You might also feel a metallic taste in your mouth. This can be remedied by simply increase your water intake. So drink as much water as needed.

More frequent urination can also be a sign you're in ketosis. Acetoacetate acid, which is a ketone body, can be found in the urine of somebody that is in ketosis. It can also cause you to go to the bathroom more often, but this symptom goes away once your body has become accustomed to a keto diet. This is also why a keto diet can cause you to become more thirsty.

You may notice that the smell of your breath has changed, this is what is known as keto breath. Not everyone eating a ketogenic diet experiences keto breath. Keto breath is caused by a ketone body called acetone escaping the body through your breath. It can makes your breath smell fruity. The smell of acetone can also be smelt in sweat during vigorous activity. But fear not, as this smell is only temporary and will fade away once your body grows accustomed to a keto diet and will stop ketones leaking into your breath and sweat. In rare cases the bad breath does not go away, here are some possible solutions than will help you if you run into this issue.

- **Drink enough fluids.** A common symptom of ketosis is a dry mouth, which means your have less saliva in your mouth to wash away bacteria. This can make the issue of bad breath worse so be sure to drink plenty of fluids and stay hydrated.

- **Maintain Oral Hygiene.** Unfortunately, brushing your teeth regularly will not solve the issue of keto breath because the smell actually comes from the lungs and not the mouth. But it can at least help mask the smell and stop it from mixing with other smells.

- **Reduce the degree of ketosis.** If the smell does not go away in a month and it's really an issue for you then you can reduce the degree of ketosis by eating more carbs. 50 – 70 grams of carbs is enough to knock you out of ketosis.

You will experience less hunger. This is because your body will become better at getting it's fuel from fat stores. People often feel great and full of energy only eating one or two meals a day, and may find themselves doing intermitted fasting without even realizing it.

Increased levels of energy is also a commonly reported symptom of being on a keto diet. When you first start a keto diet, you might actually feel like you have less energy then you usually do, this is known as the "keto flu" and it's only temporary. Once you've gotten over the keto flu you will experience a very noticeable increase in energy, some people even report feeling a sense euphoria.

MEASURING KETOSIS

There are three ways you can accurately measure ketone levels in your body. These three ways are urine strips, ketone breath analyzers and blood ketone meters.

Urine strips are the easiest and simplest way to measure ketosis. Simply dip the strip in urine and it will change colour depending on the amount of ketones in the urine. If you get a high reading, which is usually a dark purple color you'll know you're in ketosis. Ketone strips are widely available and can be found in most pharmacies or online retailer. While ketone strips are usually accurate, the results can vary a bit depending on your fluid intake. It's also important to know that when you've been on the keto diet for a while, your body becomes more efficient at reabsorbing ketones from urine back into the body. So ketone urine strips might become unreliable if you've been in ketosis for a while.

Ketone breath analyzers are another great way to measure ketone levels, although they are more expensive than urine strips. But in the long run breath analyzers will come out cheaper because they can be reused unlike urine strips. These analyzers do not provide a number for a precise level of ketones, but they give a color to indicate the general level. New models are able to connect to a computer or mobile device to give a more accurate reading.

Blood ketones meters are the most accurate method of measuring ketones. They give a precise and exact reading for the number of ketones in you blood. The downside, however is that they are generally quite expensive.

Getting into ketosis is not as black and white as you might think it is. There are varying degrees of ketosis that you should be aware of. Below 0.5 blood ketones mmol/l (millimolar) means you're not in ketosis. At this level, your body is still using glucose as it's primary source of fuel. Between 0.5 and 1.5 mmol/l is considered to be light ketosis, your body is starting to burn fat to produce ketones, but you're not all the way there yet. Between 1.5 and 3 mmol/l is optimal ketosis. This is the recommended level you should be at when you're on a keto diet. At this level, you'll see a noticeable difference in physical and mental performance and fat will be burning at a very fast rate. Over 3 mmol/l is a higher amount of ketones than necessary. At this point you won't see any more benefits over the 1.5-3 level. Higher than 3 mmol/l could mean you're not getting enough food, this is know as starvation ketosis and can be quite a dangerous situation for type 1 diabetics to be in. A blood keto level above 8 mmol/l is normally impossible by just eating a keto diet. It means something wrong is going on. The most common cause for this is type 1 diabetes and severe lack of insulin. Symptoms might including vomiting and feelings of nausea. This can lead to ketoacidosis which can be fatal, immediate medical care will be needed.

The great thing about a keto diet is that you don't even have to reach optimal ketosis to start noticing the benefits. Many benefits, such as weight loss can be experienced by just having a blood ketone level higher than 0.5 mmol/l which is very easy to achieve. Just remember that it can take weeks or months for the body to adapt to a keto diet so don't expect to see any high level benefits like increased physical and mental performance right away.

SIDE EFFECTS OF KETO

Suddenly switching your bodies primary source of energy from glucose to fat and ketones can unsurprisingly lead to some potential side effects as your body adjusts to this new way of living. Symptoms might include anything from headaches, muscle fatigue, tiredness and heart palpations. For most people, these symptoms are only mild and will fade away once the body has adjusted. Many people report feeling incredible right away, but if you don't there are ways to minimize or cure any troublesome side effects.

If you want to reduce the likelihood of any negative side effects, try gradually decreasing carb consumption for a few weeks. This slower start will give your body more time to adjust and will avoid the sudden shock of switching fuel sources. With this method the benefits of a keto diet will come through more slowly, but this might be better for you if you're worried about any negative side effects.

If you want all the benefits keto has to offer right away, then I recommend you stop consuming sugar and carbs from day one. You will likely see rapid weight loss in just a few days, even though most of that weight will be water weight. It's still highly motivating and a great way to start your keto journey.

Here is a list of some common side effects of a keto diet and how you can minimize or even completely cure them.

Keto Flu – One of the most common symptoms people experience when fist starting their keto journey. You know you have the keto flu if you experience any of these symptoms.

- Headache
- Dizziness
- Fatigue
- Nausea
- Lack of energy
- Brain fog
- Easily irritated

These are the initial symptoms and will usually disappear within a week or two, depending on how fast your body adapts to a keto diet and the increased levels of fat burning that comes with it. The reason why people get the keto flu is because foods with high a concentration of carbohydrates result in water retention in the body. When you switch to a keto diet you're not consuming carbohydrates which results in a lot of this excess fluid being lost. This loss of fluid often results in dehydration and salt depletion before your body adapts.

Thankfully, reducing or even eliminating these symptoms is quite easy. Simply make sure you're getting enough water and salt. An easy and simple way to do this is to drink a cup of broth, 1 or 2 times a day.

Leg Cramps – Leg cramps are not that common, but they can still occur when switching diets. This is only a minor issue but can be quite painful. Leg cramps are a side effect of losing too many minerals, specifically magnesium due to increased levels of urination. If you're suffering from leg cramps, be sure to drink more fluids as this will reduce the loss of magnesium. If drinking more fluids isn't helping you can try taking magnesium supplements. But if neither of these methods work, it might be a good idea to reduce your level of ketosis by introducing back some carbohydrates to you diet.

Constipation – Another possible side effect that can happen when you switch diets as your digestive system needs time to adapt. This is mainly caused by dehydration so be sure to drink a lot of fluids if you're experiencing constipation. When you're dehydrated, the body absorbs more water from the colon, this results in the contents getting dryer and harder, which results in constipation.

You will also want to consider adding more vegetables and fiber to your diet. Getting enough high quality fiber into your diet is always important, even when you're on a keto diet. Fiber helps keep the intestines moving and reduces the risk of constipation. Getting enough fiber on a low carb diet like the keto diet may prove to be challenging, as many sources of fiber are avoided. But eating non-starchy vegetables, like spinach, avocado's or asparagus can prove to very helpful in getting fiber into your diet. Another way to get some more fiber into your diet is to eat psyllium seed husks, they are completely carb free so they're a perfect option for someone on a keto diet.

Heart Palpitations – An elevated heart rate is a common experience people go through on their first few week on a low carb diet like keto. This is normal and is nothing to worry about. The most common reason for this is dehydration and lack of salt. The reduced amount of fluids circulating in the blood stream causes the heart to beat a bit harder and faster in order to maintain blood pressure. A quick and easy cure to this is to just drink more fluids and be sure to get enough salts.

If you find that drinking more water and taking more salt does not eliminate heart palpitations, then it could be the result of stress hormones released into the blood stream to maintain blood sugar levels. Fortunately, this is only temporary and will go away as your body becomes accustomed to getting its energy from burning fats.

In the unlikely situation that heart palpitations do not go away after one or two week, try slightly increasing your carbohydrate intake.

If you're on medication for diabetes or high blood pressure, avoiding carbohydrates that increase your blood pressure will lower your need for medication. Taking the same dosage of insulin prior to going on a keto diet can actually cause low blood pressure, which can also be a cause of heart palpitation.

Reduced Physical Performance – For the first one or two week on a keto diet, you'll more than likely suffer from reduced physical performance. You may be thinking to yourself "What gives, isn't my physical performance supposed to increase?". Rest assured it will, as well as your mental performance. There are two main reasons why you might experience reduced physical performance early on in the keto diet.

- **Lack of fluids.** Dehydration is a common symptom early on into the keto diet and it's the number one cause for many additional symptoms associated with a keto diet. Drink a glass of water with half a teaspoon of salt 30 to 60 minutes before exercising. You'll find this will make a huge difference in you physical performance.

- **The body adapts slowly.** Your body has been using glucose as its main source of energy for almost its entire life, so of course it's going to take time to switch from glucose to burning fat and ketones. It might take weeks or even a few months until your body has completely adapted to a keto diet and becomes a fat burning machine. Your body will adapt faster if you perform rigorous exercise while on a keto diet.

Temporary Hair Loss – Temporary hair loss can happen for a variety of reasons, one of them is when there's a big dietary change. Hair loss is especially common when on a diet that severely restrict calories, like a starvation diet. But it can occasionally occur on a keto diet. If it does happen, then it will usually be between 3 and 6 months after starting a new diet, at which point you'll notice and increased amount of hair shedding. But there's some good news. Dietary related hair loss is only a temporary phenomenon and the hair loss is very mild. After a few months on a keto diet your hair follicles will start to grow new hair and once all your hair regrows back, it will be as thick as ever before.

To understand why dietary changes can cause hair loss we need to understand how hair grows. Every hair stand on you head grows for about 2 to 3 years at a time. After which it stops growing for about three months. Then a new hair starts to grow in that same follicle, pushing the old hair strand out. So in reality, you're losing hair every day, but because the hair strands are unsynchronized this is not very noticeable. You always going to have the same number of hair stands on your scalp.

Stress is a leading factor when it comes to hair loss. When the body experiences significant stress, more hair strands then usual enter the resting phase at the same time. There are many reasons this can happen, for example:

- Diseases
- Starvation, which includes calorie restrictive diets.
- Pregnancy
- Phycological Stress
- Breast Feeding
- Physically exhausting exercise
- Big dietary changes

So what do you do if you're suffering from hair loss? If there was an obvious trigger 3 to 6 months before the hair loss started taking place, you don't really have to do anything as this side effect is only temporary. Unfortunately, you can't stop hair loss once it's happening because the resting hairs will fall out no matter what you do. So the best thing you can do is to just carry on eating on a nutritional keto diet and wait it out.

It's important to note hair loss because of a keto diet is very rare and most people never reported any issues with hair loss. Most people who lose hair on a keto diet do so because they're following the diet wrong. The keto diet is a low carb, high fat diet. Not a low carb low, low fat diet. You should be eating enough fat so that you don't feel hungry. It's also helpful to try to reduce other sources of stress. Be sure to sleep well and treat yourself well.

High Cholesterol – You may be thinking why high cholesterol is listed a negative side effect, after all isn't a keto diet supposed to help with cholesterol? Actually, it does! Going on a keto diet does indeed slightly increase your cholesterol, but this is a good thing as it increased high-density lipoprotein (HDP), also known as the good cholesterol. This leads to lower risk of heart disease.

KETO DIET AND ALCOHOL

When somebody is on a keto diet or any low carb diet, they need much less alcohol to become intoxicated. This is an important fact to remember, because you don't want to be drinking as much as you would normally drink prior to going on a keto diet. You'll probably only need half the usual amount to enjoy yourself. So not only will a keto diet make you lose weight, increase physical performance and increase mental performance, but it will also save you money at the bar! It's a win – win!

The reason for why low carb diets makes you more prone to intoxication is still unclear. It might be because the liver is too busy producing ketones and so there's less of a capacity to break down alcohol. Another reason could be because alcohol and sugar are broken down the same way in the liver. So eating less sugar would make your liver less adapted to breaking down alcohol, similar to how drinking less alcohol would.

When drinking alcohol on a keto diet, moderation is key. For someone that has a healthy liver and is at a healthy weight, the occasional low carb alcoholic drink is not going to do you any harm. Drinking too much however will slow down the effects of ketosis, including the slowing down of weight loss. If you notice you're not losing weight on a keto diet, it's recommended to just remove alcohol from your diet completely.

Many studies have shown that alcohol consumption when graphed against a morality curves in a J shape. Non-alcohol drinkers have a slightly higher morality risk than moderate drinkers, while heavy drinkers have the highest risk out of them all. It has been noted that those that drink heavily have problems with blood sugar regulation and form a sever addiction to carbohydrates. The body becomes desperate for quick sources of sugar to the brain, and alcohol is one of the fastest. Whether you drink alcohol or not on a keto diet is honestly up to you and how much willpower you have. Can you stop drinking after one or two drinks max? If you can't then it's recommended you steer clear of alcohol, as it will only get in the way of achieving ketosis.

People have experienced that going on a keto diet has reduced their cravings for alcohol and sugar greatly. This is because the diet even outs blood sugar fluctuations. Once you get past the carb addiction and your body becomes a fat burning machine, your body gains access to other sources of fuel by burning fats. So it's no longer dependent on carbohydrates and ethanol. Because a keto diet is so satisfying, the alcohol cravings subside.

The keto diet may even help alcohol detox. Detox means cleaning of the blood, which is mainly done by removing impurities from the liver. A clinical trial by The US National Institute on Alcohol Abuse and Alcoholism investigates the use of a keto diet during detox for alcohol. The results suggests that the keto diet could prove to be a promising supplementary intervention for alcohol disorders. Dr Wiers, the principle investigator has said "We will test if the ketogenic diet has an effect on withdrawal symptoms, craving, alcohol cue-induced brain reactivity and sleep quality". If it does, then the keto diet would prove to be very effective therapy for alcoholics that what to quit, she says.

In summary, drink alcohol in moderation when you're on the keto diet. If you see that you're not losing any weight go completely off it. Be aware that alcohol can trigger cravings for carbs if you drink too much. Also be aware that while on the keto diet your body will be more susceptible to becoming intoxicated. And definitely don't drink or drive, whether your on a keto diet or not.

HOW TO EAT MORE FAT

A keto diet needs to be high in fat as that's going to be the body's main source of energy. Fat is very filling so you certainly won't go hungry on a keto diet. Many people assume fat is bad, but fear not! Natural fat is good for you. Getting enough fat in your diet can be quite the challenge when you're starting the keto diet, after all most people have been avoiding it on a high carb diet. In this chapter you will learn how to get fats into your diet and what the best kinds of fat are.

Start out with whole full fat ingredients. No more avoiding high fat products, instead you want to be avoiding low fat and fat free products. Banish any item labeled low fat or fat free from your pantry and refrigerator. Say goodbye to artificial creamers, egg beaters and low-fat peanut butter. Forget about nonfat and low fat dairy products. Next time you go grocery shopping, you want to be on the lookout for fat rich, healthy whole foods like eggs or avocado. Natural fat is your best friend. Fatty cuts of meat can be a cheaper and more flavorful alternative to lean cuts. If you enjoy fish, salmon and sardines can be a wonderful addition to your diet. They're high in protein and contain plenty of healthy fats.

Next time you're cooking, instead of using oil you can use tasty natural fats like butter. Fats can change the taste of a dish and add variety to your meals. For example, you can top green beans with some butter for a warm, familiar taste. Alternatively you could sauté them in some peanut oil and top it off with sesame oil for a delicious, Asian inspired meal.

Try experimenting with different combinations and see what brings out the flavor you like best. Some examples of healthy cooking fats are:

- Olive Oil
- Coconut Oil
- Butter
- Lard or other animal fat
- Avocado Oil
- Peanut Oil or other nut oil
- Sesame Oil

No matter what meal you have, you can top it off with some high fat oil, dressing, sauces or butter. There are many fat rich sauces and dressings to choose from, mayo, gravy, hollandaise, sour cream. Choose whatever one you like.

You can also garnish your meals with some high fat foods. Garnishes like cheese, olives, seeds, cured meat, avocado and nuts make great high fat garnishing options. These whole foods add nutrients, flavor and most importantly, a whole lot of healthy fat! You can sprinkle these onto any dish. Cheese is a wonderful option to pack in more fat to your diet. It can work as an appetizer, dessert or a topping. If you're looking for an all in one fatty food, I recommended giving cheese a try.

If you're a coffee or tea addict, good news! You can turn your favorite hot beverage into a source of healthy fat. Melting butter or coconut oil into coffee is quick and easy. Topping it off with whipped cream can work too. This warm shot of fat can be drank as breakfast and is a great way to get some fat to start the day.

Snacking in general should be avoided, but if you find yourself too hungry due to lack of fats, there are plenty of high fat snacks that are easy to prepare. Like eggs, olives, cheese and avocado's. More information on fatty snacks can be found in the chapter, How To Get Into Ketosis.

You might be used to getting dessert after dinner, but it's recommended to skip it entirely when on a keto diet. But if you do decided to treat yourself, try looking for recipes that are low in sugar and high in fat. A personal favorite is unsweetened heavy whipped cream with raspberry.

So exactly how much fat should you be eating? When you're on a low carb diet like keto, the trick is to fuel your bodies energy needs with fat by cutting on carbohydrates. You will want to eat enough fat in your meals so that you're not hungry for at least the next 5 hours. You should aim to feel satisfied, not overly fed.

When you first start your keto journey, you might find that some high fat foods taste too rich. You must be patient. Your body takes time to transition from a high carb diet to a low carb, high fat diet. Both your body and taste buds will adjust to the keto diet. Focus on eating enough fat to avoid hunger and give yourself time for your body to adjust and eventually you'll become a fat burning machine. Once you've found the perfect balance, your hunger goes away as your body gains easy access to a plethora of fat stores, previously locked away by a high carb diet.

If your aim with a keto diet is to lose weight, focus on eating just enough fat so that you're not hungry. This will allow your body to burn it's internal fat stores instead of any extra fat. Doing this will greatly accelerate the rate of weight loss. But don't go too far with this. If you're hungry, get some more fat into your diet instead of caving into carbs. Once you've reached your ideal weight you no longer have the amount of internal fat stores in your body to fuel you energy needs during the day. When this happens, you need to tune into you bodies hunger signals. You do this by gradually adding more fat into your diet until you've found the ideal balance of weight maintenance without going hungry. The amount of fat needed to maintain weight is going to vary from person to person, as people have different levels of metabolism. So do some experimenting.

A trick to minimizing hunger is to make sure you're consuming the right amount of protein.

This will happen naturally for most people. If you can't stop your hunger by adding more fat to your diet, or if you're having some trouble reaching your ideal weight goal, take a look at how much protein you're including in your diet. The amount of protein needed varies from person to person, but the general rule is that you should be eating 1 gram of protein per kilogram of body weight. But, if you're an active individual and your aim is to build muscle you should be consuming more protein then that.

FOODS TO EAT

This chapter will go into more detail about specific foods you should eat on a keto diet. All foods listed here are low in carbs and are packed with healthy fats.

Seafoods

Seafood play an important role in keto diets. Salmon and other fish are rich in vitamin B, potassium and selenium. Most importantly, they're almost completely carb free.

Carbs in different species of shellfish can vary. For example, shrimp and most crabs contain no carbs, but other types of shellfish do. Here are some shellfish that can be included into your keto diet. Take into account the amount of carbs and try to keep you daily intake less than 20g. The carbs are listed for 100g servings.

- Clams – 5g
- Oysters – 4g
- Mussels – 7g
- Squid – 3g
- Octopus- 4g

Sardines, salmon, mackerel and other fatty fish all are packed with omega 3 fats, which have been linked to a decreased risk of heart disease and improved mental wellbeing. Try to consume at least two servings of seafood on a weekly basis.

Cheese

It's nutritional, delicious and it's a keto dieters best friend. There are hundreds of different types of cheese, all with varying tastes. Thankfully all them are very low in carbs and high in fat, making them the perfect food for a keto diet.

28g of cheddar cheese contains only 1g of carbs and a whopping 7g of protein. Cheese is high in saturated fats, which is known to decrease the risk of heart disease. It also contains conjugated linoleic acid, which is a fat that's been linked to weight loss. In addition to all of this, cheese has also been linked to reducing muscle deterioration due to ageing. A 12 week study done on elderly adults found that those who ate 7g of ricotta cheese a day showed an increase in muscle mass and muscle strength for the duration of the study.

Meat and Poultry

One of the staples of a keto diet, meat and poultry contain almost no carbs and are rich in vitamin B and essential minerals like potassium, zinc and selenium. They're also your number one source for protein. If possible, try selecting grass fed meat, as animals that are fed on grass have been shown to produce meat with higher amounts of omega 3 fats, antioxidants and conjugated linoleic acid than animals fed on grain.

Avocados

Avocados are one of the healthiest foods a person can eat and they're very low in carbs. 100 grams of avocado contains only 9 grams of carbs, but 7 of these carbs are fiber, so the net carbs is only 2 grams. Avocados are packed with vitamins and minerals, including potassium. Which is good news because it's been shown that a higher intake of potassium can make it easier to transition to a ketogenic diet. Avocados also contain many good fats that help improve cholesterol and triglyceride levels.

Low Carb Vegetables

Non starchy vegetables are low in carbs and packed with healthy nutrients like vitamin C and several essential minerals. Vegetables are also a good source of fiber, a type of carbohydrate that your body doesn't absorb. This is why fiber is subtracted from your carbohydrate count. Most vegetables are low in carbs, but there are a few you need to look out for. Starchy vegetables are high in carbs and include foods like potatoes, beets or yams. Vegetables also contain antioxidants that help protect against free radicals.

Low carb veggies make a great staple for keto diets. You can substitute foods like rice or mashed potatoes for cauliflower. Instead of spaghetti noodles, you can have "zoodles", which are created from zucchini and spaghetti squash. Here's a list of low carb veggies that make a great addition to a keto diet. The carb count is listed per 100 grams

- Seaweed – 0.1 grams
- Mushrooms – 0.3 grams
- Broccoli – 0.4 grams
- Cress – 0.5 grams
- Bok Choy – 0.6 grams
- Spinach – 0.9 grams
- Zucchini – 1.6 grams

Nuts and Seeds

Nuts and seeds are high in healthy fats and low in carbs. Frequent nut consumption has been linked to a reduced risk of heart disease and certain cancers. Nuts and seeds are high in fiber, which will help you feel full and helps with bowel movement. However, not all nuts are necessarily low in carbs, here is a list of popular nuts and seeds. The carb count is the net carb, meaning it's been subtracted by the amount of fiber. The carb count is for 28 grams, or 1 ounce.

- Walnuts – 2 grams
- Flax Seeds – 0 grams
- Cashews – 8 grams
- Pumpkin Seed – 4 grams
- Sesame Seed – 3 grams
- Pistachio – 5 grams
- Almonds – 3 grams
- Pecans – 1 gram
- Brazil Nuts – 1 gram

Eggs

Eggs are considered to be a superfood to many. They're highly nutritious and one large egg contains less than 1 gram of carbs, making it ideal for a keto diet. Eating the entire egg is preferable, as most of the eggs nutrients are in the yolk. Eggs are high in cholesterol, but they don't raise blood cholesterol levels in most people, in fact they've been known to reduce the risk of heart disease.

FOODS TO AVOID

When you're on a keto diet, you want to fuel your body with fats and protein instead of carbs. So naturally you want to avoid foods with high carb contents. This chapter will list foods that will slow down ketosis. These are foods that you absolutely want to avoid.

Grains

Grains are high in carbs so they should be avoided at all costs, even whole grains. Here is a list of grains and carb count per cup.

- Wheat – 15 grams
- Oats – 26 grams
- Barley – 44 grams
- Quinoa – 39 grams
- Corn – 32 grams
- Rice – 45 grams
- Rye – 15 grams

Beans and Legumes

Beans and legumes may be healthy for other diets, but they're high in carbs so should be avoided on a keto diet. Here is a list of beans and legumes. As well as their carb count per cup.

- Kidney Beans – 18.5 grams
- Lentils – 18 grams
- Green Peas – 14 grams
- Lima Beans – 19 grams
- Chickpeas – 20 grams

Most Fruits

While fruits are healthy, most of them contain a lot of carbs and sugar. But there are fruits out there that have low carb and sugar content. Fruits such as blueberries, blackberries and raspberries can be eaten on a keto diet sparingly. Here are a list of fruits you should be avoiding

- 1 Medium Orange – 17 grams
- 1 Small Banana – 18.5 grams
- 1 Medium Apple – 22 grams
- 1 Medium Mango – 50 grams
- 1 Medium Tangerine – 12 grams
- ½ Cup of Pineapple – 18 grams
- 1 Cup of grapes 27 grams

<u>**Starchy Vegetables**</u>
Vegetables grown in the ground tend to be high in carbs. These include things like potatoes, yams and parsnips. Some ground grown foods can be eaten on occasion, like carrots. Here is a list of starchy vegetables you should avoid with a carb count per half cup of cooked vegetables.

- Yams – 19 grams
- Carrots – 6 grams
- Peas – 14 grams
- Sweet Potatoes – 14 grams
- Corn – 32 grams
- Parsnips – 15 grams
- Cherry Tomatoes – 6 grams

<u>**Sugars**</u>
In todays day and age, sugars are almost inescapable. Consuming too much sugar will kick you out of ketosis so it should be avoided at all costs.

<u>**Unhealthy Fat Foods**</u>
Even though you'll be getting most of your energy from fats, it's important to avoid unhealthy ones. Processed vegetable oils contain a lot of unhealthy fats so they should

be avoided. Here is a list of oils to avoid.

- Corn Oil
- Peanut Oil
- Sesame Oil
- Soybean Oil
- Grapeseed Oil
- Canola Oi
- Safflower Oil

Alcohol

For some people, this may be difficult to give up, but most alcoholic drinks are high in carbs and can easily knock you out of ketosis. Here are some high carb alcoholic drinks you should watch out for:

- Beer (12 fluid ounces) – 12.7 grams
- Wine (1 Glass) – 14 grams
- Cocktails – 5 grams

Sugary Beverages

It's a good idea too stay away from sweetened beverages. They hold no nutritional value and are very high in carbs.

- 1 Can Sugary Soda – 36 grams
- 1 Can Diet Soda – 0 grams (No Nutrition)
- 1 Cup Fruit Juice – 18 grams

FREQUENTLY ASKED QUESTIONS

This chapter will go over frequently asked questions about the keto diet. It presents a convenient way of getting information without having to flick through the entire book.

What Food Can I Eat?

The main thing you want to do is stay away from carbs. So foods like pasta, bread, sugars and rice should all be avoided. Some foods may surprise you with how much carbohydrates they contain, so be sure to read the label for carbohydrates.

Even vegetables can have carbs in them, but they're still a necessary part of any diet, including low carb diets like keto. That's why you're allowed to have a maximum of 20 – 30 grams of carbs a day, it's to allow wiggle room for foods that we need. More information on what kinds of foods to eat can be found in chapter 5 – How to Get Into Ketosis.

Can I Eat Too Much Fat?

Yes, it is possible to eat too much fat on a keto diet. If you want to lose weight, you still need to be eating at a caloric deficient, even on a keto diet. Eating too much fat will put you on a caloric surplus. For the average person, eating too much fat on a keto diet is extremely hard, but it's still possible.

You can find keto calculators online to calculate your macros and find out how much protein, fats and carbs you should be eating a day. You should edit the values of protein and fat with your activity level in mind. If you're very active, say you like playing sports or bodybuilding, your protein and fat requirements will be greater then the average person.

Can I Get a Heart Attack From Eating All This Fat?

It's a good question. Many people have misconceptions about fat and keto diets. There are three main fat groups that we eat. These fats are saturated fats, monounsaturated fats and polyunsaturated fats. People used to think that saturated fats were unhealthy and that there was a clear link between saturated fats and heart disease. However, it's recently been brought to light that saturated fats have no correlation with heart disease, in fact it's been discovered that saturated fats can actually improve cholesterol levels. So there's no need to feel bad about yourself you eating saturated fats.

Polyunsaturated fats are a little more trickier. Processed polyunsaturated fats are not good for us, and usually include trans fats. Too much processed polyunsaturated fats has been linked with causing heart disease so it should be avoided. But the flip side of the coin is natural polyunsaturated fats which can be found in foods like fish, they're a great way to help improve cholesterol.

Last but not least are monosaturated fats, which are known to be healthy. Olive oil is a primary example of monosaturated fats and can also lower cholesterol.

So in summary, saturated, monosaturated and natural polyunsaturated fats are healthy and can help to lower cholesterol. Avoid processed polyunsaturated fats as they have been linked to heart disease. Foods high in processed polyunsaturated fats include vegetable oil and margarine.

Do I need to count my calories?

No matter what diet you take, at the end of

the day calories do matter. The amount of calories you take all depends on what your goal is. If your goal is to lose weight then you should go on a calorie deficit. If your goal is to maintain your body weight, then you need to find the right amount of calories for your body to maintain it's weight.

With a ketogenic diet you rarely have to worry about calories because you'll be eating mostly fats and protein which will keep you feeling full for long periods of time. Calorie requirement varies from person to person. With exercise calorie requirements go up so you should be eating more to make up for the energy expended performing exercise.

How can I track my carbs?
There are plenty of website and mobile apps that you can use to track your carb intake. The most popular one would probably be MyFitnessPal, which also has a mobile app. You won't be able to track you net carbs on the app, but you can track your total carb and fiber intake. If you want to calculate your net carbs, simply subtract your total fiber intake from your total carb intake.

How long does it take to get into ketosis?

Ketosis is not something you get into immediately, it takes time for you body to adjust and enter a state of ketosis. This process can take anywhere between two to seven days. This time varies from person to person. It depends on your activity levels, body type and what kind of foods you're eating. Exercising while on a keto diet can lead your body to go into a state of ketosis faster. The less carbohydrates your eat, the faster you'll enter ketosis. Try to keep your carb intake less than 20g a day. It's also important to stay hydrated, because your body can suffer from dehydration while it's adapting to a keto diet.

How much weight will I lose?

This is entirely dependent on you. Supplementing the keto diet with exercise is one of the fastest ways you can lose weight. When you're in a state of ketosis your body will constantly be burning fat to supply your body with energy in the form of ketones. So your job will be to stay in ketosis for as long as possible. The more you substitute carbs for fat and protein in your diet, the faster you'll enter ketosis and the more weight you will lose. You might be shocked that your body has has lost weight in only a few days on a keto diet. But this weight is actually water weight, not fat. To continue losing fat requires dedication.

The keto diet makes me feel constipated, what should I do?

Constipation is fairly common in people starting a new diet. Below is a list of advice to help with constipation.

- Drink plenty of water
- Get more fiber into your diet
- Take magnesium supplements
- Eat a tablespoon of coconut oil
- Avoid nuts
- Try drinking tea of coffee

I'm feeling lethargic, what should I do?

Feeling low on energy and getting headaches is very common with people starting a keto diet. It's even been nick named the keto flu. The keto flu is caused because the body needs to urinate a lot more, which can cause dehydration if you're not drink enough water to compensate. Rehydrate yourself by drinking plenty of water with a little added salt. Salty foods like salted nuts, bacon or deli meat can be a good way of getting more salt into your diet.

I work out, should I avoid the keto diet?

When it comes to working out, there are two types of people. People who love to run, and people who love to lift weights. If you're someone that does a lot of cardio, be it running, cycling, swimming, etc. Then you don't need to worry. Studies have shown that low carb diets like keto have no negative effects on aerobic exercises.

If you lift weights then you have to be aware of your end goal. Carbohydrates do help with performance and muscle recovery when it comes to weight lifting. So there are two paths you can take, targeted ketogenic diet or cyclidic ketogenic diet.

A targeted ketogenic diet is when you're consuming just enough carbs before your workout to knock you out of ketosis. It works by supplying glycogen to your muscles for the duration of the workouts. After your workout you will go back into ketosis because you've used up all your glycogen stores doing exercise.

A cyclic ketogenic diet is a bit more advanced

than a targeted ketogenic diet, it's not recommended for anyone that's new to a keto diet or training. It's more for bodybuilders or athletes that want to stay on a keto diet while still building muscle. This method involves staying on a keto diet for a certain period, usually five days. After that period you replenish your bodies glycogen stores by eating enough carbs to last your body five days of intense workouts. What you're essentially doing is packing your body with glycogen in order to fuel your training regime. Then by the time your training is finished your glycogen stores will be depleted and you're back into ketosis.

Can I drink alcohol on a keto diet?
Alcohol can be consumed on a keto diet, but you need to be extra vigilant. Most alcoholic drinks are packed with carbs. Wine, beer and cocktails all contain carbohydrates. Your best bet would be clear liquor, as these have the lowest carb contents.

My weight loss has stalled, what should I do?
Weight loss plateaus happen to everyone. There are a number of things that could be causing the problem, so you may need to try

many methods to help you. Here's a list of things you can try if you've stalled on weight loss.

- Stop eating gluten
- Cut out dairy from your diet
- Reduce your carb intake even further
- Watch out for foods with hidden carbs
- Stop eating nuts
- Avoid artificial sweeteners
- Stop eating processed foods
- Include more fat into your diet.

Should I take any supplements for a keto diet?

You don't need to take any supplements to go into ketosis, as it's a natural process that your body can do on it's own. But some people may suffer from symptoms when first starting the diet and may not feel well. Some supplements to ease these symptoms include:

- Multivitamins
- Magnesium Supplements
- Vitamin B Complex
- Vitamin D Supplements
- Potassium Supplements

Always consult a doctor before introducing any vitamins to your diet.

85

About the Author

Randall Colbert is a nutritional expert and self-published writer. He received his bachelor of Nutritional Sciences degree at Cornell University. His mission is to help people of all ages to develop healthy relationships with food. As a registered dietician he's passionate about how diets can effect the human body and even cure diseases.